Native American Healing Secrets

Mastering the art of Native American healing

Emma Lee Walker

TERMS AND CONDITIONS

LEGAL NOTICE

The Publisher has strived to be as accurate and complete as possible in the creation of this report, notwithstanding the fact that he does not warrant or represent at any time that the contents within are accurate due to the rapidly changing nature of the Internet.

While all attempts have been made to verify information provided in this publication, the Publisher assumes no responsibility for errors, omissions, or contrary interpretation of the subject Matter herein. Any perceived slights of specific persons, peoples, or organizations are unintentional.

In practical advice books, like anything else in life, there are no guarantees of income made. Readers are cautioned to reply on their own judgment about their individual circumstances to act accordingly.

This book is not intended for use as a source of legal, business, accounting or financial advice. All readers are advised to seek services of competent professionals in legal, business, accounting and finance fields.

You are encouraged to print this book for easy reading.

TABLE OF CONTENTS

FOREWORD

A lot of healing practices and spiritual ceremonials that are being practiced nowadays by healing practitioners and metaphysical groups have been acquired from traditions that initiated from assorted Native American tribes.

History suggests that every tribe would have one or more elders who were trained in the healing arts. These people would serve as herbalists, healers, and spirit communicators. The responsibilities and types of healing arts and spiritual ceremonials performed would by nature vary from tribe to tribe.

Chapter 1: Animal Medicine And Totems

Synopsis

Native American rituals and practices are rooted in association with all facets of life and the Great Spirit (God). Consequently, the Native American exercise of "animal medicine" covers an awareness that conveys itself when a particular animal crosses our path.

The word "medicine" in Native American use and in the tradition of animal medicine concerns the healing facets that a certain animal brings to our consciousness. This would imply anything that defends, strengthens, restores, empowers, or repairs the spiritual body, in addition to the physical body.

The Animals

Once we're aware of what a particular animal represents, then we may take the necessary steps to produce changes in our life according to that cognizance.

In the accompanying illustrations, you'll notice that there's reference to "crow individuals," "spider individuals" or "ant individuals." This is because the individual who sees the animal medicine is named for the animal while they're becoming cognizant or when they're in the middle of altering a behavior due to the cognizance.

Illustration 1 - Crow medicine: In Cherokee: (koga nvwati)

Crow

"Crow medicine" has the power to shape-shift. This implies they may be 2 places at one time. When "crow individuals" see or listen to crow medicine, it brings a cognizance that they're able to be in 2 places at whatever given time.

This might be presenting a lecture and jointly talking to you through this book. It's being on the radio and talking to you at the same time through this book. I may likewise be working with a person and at the same time talking through the book. It may be a speaking to you by writing a book and through a radio show at the same time.

This may present confirmation that being versatile will help someone reach more individuals at the same time and that someone is doing what they love.
And some of the times Crow medicine reinforces shape-shifting when someone finds themselves in a mode of sluggishness or when they haven't been working as diligently as they ought to be. Crow medicine brings someone back to getting his or her work accomplished.

Illustration 2 - spider medicine: In Cherokee: (kananesgi nvwati)

Spider

When people have been dillydallying on a few projects, spider medicine can help. When you see a huge spider crawling across the floor it may be a sign. This can mean that spider medicine means business and it unquestionably wants you to see it! One versed in spider medicine will know exactly what the "spider medicine" delineated.

Spider Medicine constitutes creative thinking. Its eight legs comprise the four winds of change and the four directions on the medicine wheel. Its torso is in the shape of an eight, which exemplifies numberless possibilities. "Spider individuals" have to look beyond the web of fantasy of the physical world and look on the far side of the horizon to additional dimensions.

It signifies, "wake up and become originative. You've got a lot to tell. Think, produce, think, and create." Needless to say, spider medicine can say get back to your office and begin weaving fresh patterns for your life. If you see the spider medicine (the spider) takes it somewhere where she will be safe and comfy. Then welcome her to visit you another time when you start getting off track.

Illustration 3 - ant medicine: In Cherokee: (tsosudali nvwati)

Ants

Ants have strength and determination. Also, they are team players.

Ant medicine demands our attention, patience, persistence and endurance. Think of your level of patience and the nature of the topic at hand. "Ant individuals" recognize that there's light at the end of the tunnel. It likewise says, "What is yours will come to you."

It will tell you that with trust and patience, God will provide. If you've realized that you are working really hard and not seeing the fruits of your labor don't worry. Frankly, there are no worries with ant medicine present. It likewise serves as a gentle reminder that patience does have its advantages.

Do some research on what animals represent what type of healing, and then you may use totem poles of those animals to draw the healing powers of that animal whenever you look at it.

Chapter 2: Sweat Lodge

Synopsis

The sweat lodge is a Native American custom where people get into a dome-shaped dwelling to go through a sauna-like environment. The lodge itself is commonly a wooden-framed structure made from tree limbs. Hot rocks are laid inside an earthen-dug pit set in the center of this man-made enclosure.

Water is sporadically poured over the heated rocks to produce a hot and steamy room. The sweat ceremonial is meant as a spiritual reunion with the creator and a venerating connection to the earth itself as much as it's meant for purging toxins from the physical body.

Purging Things From The Body

Mental mending - The sweat lodge ceremonial presents its participants the chance to free their minds of distractions, offering lucidity.

Spiritual mending - The sweat lodge ceremonial provides a place for introspection and connection to the planet and the spirit domain.

Physical Healing:

The sweat lodge ceremonial presents anti-bacterial and wound-healing advantages. An entire Medical Review of the health advantages and risks of Native American sweat lodges were published by the Indian Health Service in 1998.

The heat of a sweat lodge is able to raise core body temperature, producing what may be called a "temporary fever." In a sauna at 80 degrees Centigrade (C), grownups raise their rectal temperature about 1 degree C after a half-hour. There's increasing evidence that mild to moderate pinnacles of temperature may heighten particular and nonspecific immunity.

Febrile temperatures have been demonstrated to advance the migration of neutrophiles, the production of antibacterial matters by leukocytes, and the antiviral action of interferon. An experiment with mice contaminated with herpes supplies a dramatic illustration of bettered host defenses: increasing their core temperature by 2 degrees Centigrade bettered their survival rate from 0% to 100%.

Anti-cancer:
Hyperthermia seems to be a promising modality for cancer handling when blended with radiotherapy or chemotherapy, though the experimental body temperatures (41-45 degrees C) are well above those received in a sweat lodge.

Yet there might likewise be anti-cancer benefits to elevating body temperature to the febrile range. Elevated temperatures have been evidenced to retard the proliferation of particular tumor cells, increase the antitumor action of interferon and interleukins, and heighten the killing efficiency of particular cytotoxic t-lymphocytes

Detoxification:

The idea that injurious "toxins" may be eliminated from the body by sweating is a popular one, as demonstrated by these quotes from publications designated for the general public: "Sweating is among our most crucial mechanisms of natural healing, as it allows the body to free itself of unwanted materials, "Impurities in a lot of body organs are purged out as the capillaries dilate and the heart step-ups its pace, "'Heat stress'...is really effective in freeing fat-stored toxins from the cells.

While there's no doubt that sweat glands are excretory organs, the clinical implication of human sweat as an excretory pathway for particular substances has got little scientific scrutiny.

However there may be dangers to this type of treatment. Make sure that you check with a doctor first and pay attention to the cues your body is giving you.

Chapter 3: Dreamcatchers

Synopsis

The earliest dreamcatchers (sacred hoops) were crafted for youngsters to protect them from nightmares. Dreamcatchers were originally made by the youngsters of the Native American Kiowa and Cherokee tribes.

Dreamcatchers constitute a spider's web with a hole in the centre. The web catches the foul dreams which melt in the sunshine, and the beneficial dreams pass through the center hole and travel down the feather suspended from the center.

Sleep Healing

The legend of the Native American dreamcatcher deviates somewhat from tribe to tribe, however the basic theme or aim was to let good dreams slip through the web and into the sleeper during the nighttime while the foul dreams were caught up in the web and would be perished at break of day light. The Lakota Legend has the opposing notion that the web will catch your great ideas and the bad ones will pass through the hole.

Sacred Hoops

The earliest dreamcatchers, normally called Sacred Hoops, were crafted by parents to protect their youngsters from nightmares. Newborns were presented charms that were wound in the form of spider webs to protect their dreams so their innocence wouldn't be harmed by the pranksters of the night. The dream catcher charm is hung from the hoop on the cradle.

How They Were Made

Dreamcatcher hoops were in the beginning made out of willow and covered up with sage, the web was made from deer tendon. Modern dreamcatchers are constructed with wood or metal wound in leather strips, artificial tendon replace the now forbidden utilization of deer tendon. The decoration of the web along with the form, size and colors utilized is left to the artisan's imagination. Feathers bound to the dreamcatcher are meant to assist the flight of great dreams.

The Story of the Dreamcatcher

From The Chippewa

A spider was softly spinning his web in his own place. It was alongside the sleeping space of Nokomis, the grandma. Every day,

Nokomis watched the spider at work, softly spinning away.

One day as she was looking at him, her grandson entered. "Nokomis-iya!" he cried, peeking at the spider. He stamped over to the spider, gathered up a shoe and went to hit it.

"No-keegwa," the old lady whispered, "don't harm him."

"Nokomis, why do you protect the spider?" Enquired the little boy.

The old lady smiled, but didn't answer. Once the boy left, the spider went to the old lady and thanked her for sparing his life. He stated to her, "For numerous days you've watched me spin and weave my web. You've admired my work. In return for sparing my life, I'll give you a gift."

He smiled his particular spider smile and moved away, spinning as he exited.

Before long the moon glistened on a magical silverish web moving softly in the window. "See how I spin?" he stated. "See and learn, for every web will snare foul dreams.

Only great dreams will run through the little hole. This is my present to you. Use it so that only great dreams will be recalled. The foul dreams will get hopelessly entangled in the web."

This is an ancient legend, as dreams will never cease, hang this dream net above your bed, dream on, and be at peace.

CHAPTER 4: FEATHERS IN HEALING

SYNOPSIS

Feathers are our connectedness to the "air" forces; air being among the four elements. The remaining 3 elements are water, fire, and earth. A healer may incorporate the utilization of feathers in assorted ways. The feather is valuable in cleaning auras. The healer might breathe through the feather during a toning session. Chanting sounds through a feather on client's body may evoke a potent healing.

Gifts From Feathered Friends

The 4 basic elements (occasionally called "temperaments") are air, earth, fire, and water. Comprehending what every element represents helps us assess where our individual strengths and weaknesses are.

Healers have discovered that centering on the elements may often be helpful when looking for what class of treatments would best address our troubles.

- Air exemplifies intellect, mental intent, and association to universal life force.
- Earth exemplifies grounding, basis of life, substance, association to life path, and family bases.
- Fire constitutes power, tool for transformation, association to personal energy, and inner force.
- Water constitutes emotional release, hunch, and interior reflection.

Different sorts of feathers are utilized depending on the requirement of the client.

Turkey feathers are marvelous for cleaning auras, the bowels, and the total gastrointestinal tract. Turkey totem constitutes a time of harvest and blessings.

Turkey is rather a little like buffalo- really sacred. It's one that gives unconditionally. If you keep an eye on a wild turkey and watch you'll find additional foods to eat. The plumes have been utilized to make caps for ceremonials as well as to keep rain off. Nearly every part of the turkey may be utilized for one thing or another and naturally the bird is likewise a food source. To the Cherokee the turkey was as hallowed as the eagle if not more so. Turkeys instruct adaptivity for that is what has assisted them in surviving the devastation of their forest.

They're nest sharers with numerous hens maintaining eggs in the same nest and tending to them. This assures a greater survival for all the chicks. It teaches being strong through being in the flock and letting others assist you in not only discovering food but also raising your offspring and being a part of the whole.

Cardinal feathers returns vitality to blood conditions and boosts energy states in anemia sufferers. Meanings and Messages: self-acknowledgement, life-blood, repaired energy, and responsibility towards loved ones

The cardinal, a red finch, is well recognized among other birds. Cardinals likewise tend to stay put for all seasons so are easy to spot year round. As a totem they inject vitality or serve as a reminder that life force is lacking.

What is your energy state right now? You might likewise need to brighten up a drab wardrobe with some color.

Cardinals will sing loudly to alert danger, for this reason a cardinal sighting may be a signal to be on alert for potential trouble. The cardinal is family-oriented. The male assists with feeding and protecting the fledglings. Ask yourself if loved ones are at risk or need extra care.

Down feathers are great for healing skin conditions, perking up the sense of touch, and calms mental chatter.

Educate yourself to perform healing by grounding, associating to your higher self, centering and protecting your energy.

Select an appropriate feather- you might want to keep one specifically for this use. If you wish to link to a particular bird energy and you don't have a feather from that bird then select a feather with a like coloring and visualize the bird you wish to link with as you work with it.

Spend a minute connecting to the bird energy by envisioning it and holding the feather between your hands. Now trigger your feather by breathing on it. This procedure may all be done in advance.

If you utilize the feather in the aura work all around the other individual smoothing downward from head to foot. It's best if they're standing or sitting. Include beneath their arms and beneath their feet.

Pay extra attention to any dense, gummy areas where the feather doesn't wish to flow. Feathers are like antennae and may guide you to the afflicted spots. Avoid putting owl feathers onto the body; they may drive the trouble further in.

CHAPTER 5: PRAYER TIES

SYNOPSIS

Native Americans provide prayer ties to The Great Spirit in exchange for blessings. Nevertheless, you don't have to be Native American to take up this earth-centered ritual of making and utilizing prayer ties as a purpose tool for prayer or healing.

Offerings

Prayer ties are spiritual tools produced to be a physical representation and bearers of the energy of a prayer. Building Prayer Ties is a ceremony inside itself. The procedure ought to be done with a great deal of reverence and respect.

The ceremonial and the procedure are different with a lot of elders or teachers. Be cognizant that there are a lot of forms and you might envision and design ones of your own.

Cut about a 2-½" x 2-½" square piece of natural cloth. The color may be any color you pick out that represents the prayer you're making. Tied bundles strung up together frequently have four colors constituting the unity of the 4 directions.

If you tie the bundles to a hallowed tree or other relation you might wish to tie downy feathers with them so that once the wind blows it carries your prayer above.

Materials

As you collect your materials, keep your intent centered on honoring the materials, plants or herbs you choose to utilize.

- Colored cotton cloth cut in 2-½" x 2-½" squares. (Yellow, red, black, white, blue, purple, green.)
- Fresh cedar tree branches (the green ends). If you wish to add fresh cedar.
- Tobacco. Strip the spines from the leaf if you're utilizing leaf tobacco.

- Cotton string, Kite string works well as does crocheting thread
- Sage (to smudge yourself and all your provisions)

Additional sacred plants are utilized for smudging, a purification process in which a plant's aromatic smoke cleans an area of damaging energies, thoughts, feelings, and spirits. Smudging is a central element of healing prayers and ceremonies.

The most typically utilized plants are sage (not the food spice) and cedar, which chase away damaging energy, and sweet grass, which takes in favorable, healing spirits.

Ironically, the most spiritually mighty plant is tobacco, today's substance of heaviest abuse. Tobacco is the herb of prayer, put on earth by spirits to help us commune with them and nature. All tobacco utilization, ranging from ceremonial to cigarettes, ought to be treated with respect and awareness.

As you make the ties, keep your intent centered on connecting to the Creator. After you've cut the squares, take a pinch of tobacco only or a concoction of tobacco, sweet grass, sage and/or additional herbs are placed in the middle of the cloth as you state your prayer.

Then place the tobacco before of your mouth and nose and breath into it and talk about the qualities that you build with this bundle, talk about the qualities of creation and the great power that goes with it. (This might be a little pinch as it's all that's required to hold your prayer.) Your prayer is therefore mentally placed, and uttered into "tobacco" into the bundle.

Fold the fabric over, fold it once again and one more time. Pinch the bundle together; tie it at the top around the pinch of tobacco.

Placement

As you position the ties, keep your intent centered on producing a hallowed circle of protection and oneness.

Directive Color Symbolism

- East: yellow - break of day, spring, rebirthing, Great Eagle
- South: red - noon, summertime, puberty, Trickster Coyote
- West: black -afternoon, fall, harvest time, maturity, Great Bear
- North: white - evening, wintertime, ancestors and elders, hallowed white buffalo
- Blue - Father Sky, water, rain, Thunder Beings, curing energy
- Green - Mother Earth, All creation, plants, creatures, 4 seasons
- Purple - Creator, Old Ancient Ones.

CHAPTER 6: SMUDGING

SYNOPSIS

Utilizing a smudging tool is part of a lot of Native American traditions. The burning of herbs for emotional, psychic, and spiritual purgation is likewise common practice among a lot of religious, healing, and spiritual groups.

The rite of smudging may be defined as "spiritual house cleansing." In essence, the smoke attaches itself to damaging energy and as the smoke clears it takes the damaging energy with it, discharging it into a different space where it will be reformed into favorable energy.

A Few More Advantages

In a lot of traditions, smudging requires a 4 directions ceremony or prayer, which sends off particular sorts of smoke or prayers into the 4 directions. Different tribes have assorted smudging prayers that program the smoke to do a particular action, like cleansing or aiding in divination.

Generally, smudging may be used in daily life for practical intents: to restore physical, mental and emotional balance; to screen against damaging energies; to clean yourself, your magical tools and your space; and to mend you sacred space.

You may burn these common smudging herbs separately or in combination with one another. One great combination that covers all 4 magical components of air, fire, water and earth is pine resin and sage (either desert sage or white broadleaf sage). This compound is appropriate for universal use, cleansing, ceremony and ritual.

Common Herbs Used in Smudge Sticks

- Sage / White Sage
- Cedar / Pine
- Lavender
- Sweet Grass
- Mugwort
- Copal

What To Smudge

- Yourself
- Crystals
- Personal Objects
- Home / Office / Healing Space

When To Smudge Yourself

- When your spirits are low

- After being around somebody who's sick or blue
- During meditation
- If in prayer

Smudging yourself on a day-to-day basis may be really helpful in keeping yourself balanced and preserving a peaceful state of being.

But, you ought to definitely utilize smudging processes when you've been around individuals who are ill, blue, fearful, angry or broadly emotionally unbalanced; prior to meditating to produce a calm state of being; when you're feeling depressed or blue; or when you've been under much stress.

Smudging yourself is simple. If you're utilizing a smudge stick, light the smudge stick on a candle. Hold the stick in the flame till there's a lot of smoke and the stick is ablaze well.

Utilizing a feather (or feather fan) or your hand, softly fan the smoke onto your body, beginning at the top of the body and moving downwards. Get the back of your body as best you are able to. Once you're done, breathe in a little of the smoke (just a bit!) to purify your insides.

If you're utilizing a smudge pot or fire bowl and loose herbs, light the herbs till they are smoking well. Then, place the fire bowl on the ground and stand over it with your legs spread out and feet on either side.

Waver back and forth in the smoke till you've been thoroughly cleansed. Apparel is optional for this approach, and smudging in the nude is advocated for a more thorough purifying.

Again, when you're finished, inhale a bit of the smoke to purify your insides. Individuals frequently feel more relaxed, lighter and brighter following smudging.

If you're going to utilize the smudge smoke during meditation, utilize a charcoal burner or fire bowl, light the herbs and savor the scent and smoke as you meditate. Meditating with these herbs frequently produces a deeper and longer-lasting state of relaxation and reflection.

CHAPTER 7: PEACE PIPES

SYNOPSIS

Kinnick Kinnick is what a few Native Americans call a particular blend of wild-crafted herbs utilized for smoking ceremonial peace pipes. Kinnick Kinnick bears no tobacco but dried tobacco leaves are occasionally mixed in with Kinnick Kinnick prior to utilizing.

Passing The Pipe

Ceremonial utilization of tobacco by Native Americans is traditionally regarded as an offering to the spirits. Herbs utilized in Kinnick Kinnick blends are assorted. Bearberry leaf is the main herb; additional herbs in Kinnick Kinnick mixtures generally include yerba santa leaf, mullein, red willow bark, and osha root. Kinnick Kinnick is occasionally placed loose within a clay bowl or abalone shell and fired as an incense or smudge herb.

To ready kinnic kinnic, a man cut red osier dogwood stems and packed them back home where he scratched off the outer bark with a pocketknife. With the back of the knife blade, he then scratched curlicues of inner bark from the stem, and let them fall in a cloth placed over his lap.

He then made a drying rack by dividing one of the peeled stems midway down and opening the end to form a Y. The opened up portion was then woven with criss-crosses of additional split stems to form a grid, and on this he placed the scrolls of inner bark. He forced the rack into the ground diagonally, simply above a low fire, so the bark was about a foot higher up than the flames and could dry in the heat without becoming burned. In about 20 minutes the bark was toasted and crisp and could be pulverized to the consistency of a rough-cut tobacco by chafing it between the palms.

Roles of herbs generally found in Kinnick Kinnick mixtures:

- Bearberry Leaves: Purification

Bearberry is a little evergreen shrub frequently utilized as a groundcover. It's an excellent choice to provide winter interest with the tiny leaves that turn bronzy in the fall, and the little red berries that last till springtime. Bearberry is likewise useful for drought and salt-tolerant landscapes. Bearberry has peeling, red bark, a different point in its favor as a winter interest shrub. Bearberry is utilized in alternative medicine to treat bladder troubles.

- Deer Tongue: Flavor
- Mullein: Protection
- Osha Root: Power, Luck
- Red Raspberry Leaf: Throat Soother

Wild red raspberry leaves are a savory and nutritive herb. Red raspberry fruits are a familiar treat for each child who has had the opportunity to walk in the country on a hot summertime day. The leaves are flavorful and abundant, picked from early summertime till fall and merely dried till they crumble.

The resulting product is utilized for a delicious tea, either hot or iced, tinctured for diarrhea and a supportive herb for a woman's reproductive system. Red raspberry leaves are a marvelously soothing and healing remedy for a canker sore. Dampen a teaspoon of red raspberry leaves with warm water till they make a soft clump. Lay these moistened leaves onto the canker and hold it there as long as you are able to. This remedy will soothe the area and by the next day you might find that it is almost healed! This is a time-tested remedy.

- Red Willow Bark: Spirit Communicator
- Tobacco: Prayer Offering
- Yerba Santa: Sweetness

Yerba Santa leaves are traditionally utilized as a smudging herb for heightening psychic abilities, magical protection, healing, and spiritual potency. Excellent for meditation and divination, Yerba Santa, is said to be ruled by the moon. One Native American tribe rolled the leaves into balls, dehydrated it in the sun, and chewed it for a natural mouthwash.

The pipe ceremony is a hallowed ritual for linking up physical and spiritual worlds. The pipe is a connection between the earth and the sky. Nothing is more hallowed. The pipe is our prayers in physical form. Smoke turns into our words; it goes out, touches everything, and gets to be a part of all there is. The fire in the pipe is the same fire in the sunshine, which is the origin of life. The reason why tobacco is utilized to connect the worlds is that the plant's roots go far into the earth, and its smoke ascents high into the heavens.

There are assorted kinds of pipes and different utilizations for them. There are personal pipes and family pipes as well as pipes for big ceremonies. The particular stone utilized depends on the tribe's location, and assorted symbols are added to attract particular spiritual energies. Likewise, the sort of tobacco utilized depends upon tribal custom. But in spite of these differences, there are particular important similarities: The ceremony calls forth a relationship with the energies of the universe, and ultimately the Creator, and the bond made between earthly and spiritual realms isn't to be broken.

CHAPTER 8: HEALING HERBS

SYNOPSIS

Because of Native Americans' intimate relationship with nature, a lot of therapies emphasize plants' mind-body-spirit healing potential.

Plant Life

Native-American herbalism is much more composite than herbs merely serving as a plant matrix to deliver physiologically active chemicals.

First of all, because numerous plant elements affect bodily functions and bioavailability, the total remedy is considered the active agent.

Secondly, as plants are believed to possess spirit and intelligence, they're conferred with to determine their best healing relationship with patients, and permission is obtained prior to and gratitude expressed following harvesting them.

Thirdly, involved procedures are utilized to harvest herbs, considering factors like plant part (e.g., flower, stem, root, and so forth), time or season of harvest, sun exposure, and a great deal more obscure factors.

Fourthly, native herbalists utilize plants that come up in dreams, a form of communication by which the plant's spirit may guide the healer.

Lastly, the plant's healing potency is empowered by ritual ceremony, prayer, song, or chants.

CHAPTER 9: MEDICINE WHEEL

SYNOPSIS

The medicine wheel, developing from Native American traditions, is likewise referred to as Sacred Hoop. The medicine wheel constitutes the sacred circle of life, its general 4 directions, and the elements.

Animal totems serve up as guardian of every one of the directions.

The 4 animals generally represented in this role are The Bear, The Buffalo, The Eagle, and The Mouse. All the same, there are no firm rules about which animals constitute the directions of the Medicine Wheel.

All native tribes have different spirit animals and significances of the directions, encouraging us in picking out our own. Every direction of the wheel provides its own lessons, color, and animal spirit guide.

Sacred Hoop

The medicine wheel is a symbolization of symmetry and balance. During the procedure of building the wheel you'll begin to realize what areas of your life are not in balance, and where your attending is lacking and demands centering.

Continuing working with the wheel after you built it. Sit with your wheel in still meditation. Allow the wheel to help you in acquiring fresh and different perspectives.

The medicine wheel constitutes the many cycles of life. The circle is representative of life's ceaseless cycle (birth, death, rebirth). Every stone or spoke placement in the wheel centers on a different facet of living.

A personal medicine wheel may be constructed utilizing fetishes like crystals, arrowheads, seashells, feathers, animal fur/bones, and so forth. Take time to reflect on every aspect of your life (self, loved ones, relationships, life aim, community, finances, wellness, and so forth.) as you place objects inside the circle.

A medicine wheel may likewise be constructed without the utilization of objects, merely draw out your circle with colored pencils and paper. If you have the room outside for a large-scale medicine wheel and are up to the project plow ahead.

If you are able to make it large enough for you to sit inside the spaces between the spokes of the wheel after you've built it, even better!

Medicine Wheel Elements and Directions

Four Elements:
Air, Water, Fire, Earth

Four Directions:
North, East, South, West

Five Directions;
North, East, South, West, Center (Heart)

Six Directions:
North, East, South, West, Sky, Earth

Seven Directions:
North, East, South, West, Father Sky, Mother Earth, Center (Self)

Medicine wheels are constructed by laying stones in a particular pattern on the ground. Most medicine wheels follow the general pattern of having a center cairn of stones, and encompassing that would be an outer ring of stones, then there will be "spokes", or lines of rocks, emerging from the cairn.

They often look like a wagon wheel lying on its side. The wheels may be large, reaching diameters of 75 feet.

Almost all medicine wheels would have at least 2 of the 3 elements mentioned above (the center cairn, the outer ring, and the spokes), but on the far side of that there are many variations on this basic design, and every wheel is unique and has had its own style and eccentricities.

The basic deviation between different wheels are the spokes. There's no set number of spokes for a medicine wheel to have. The spokes inside each wheel are seldom evenly spaced out, or even all the equivalent length. A few medicine wheels will have one certain spoke that's significantly longer than the rest, indicating something crucial about the direction it points.

A different variation is whether the spokes begin from the center cairn and go out only to the outer ring, or whether they go past the outer ring, or whether they begin at the outer ring and go out from there.

An odd version occasionally discovered in medicine wheels is the presence of a passage, or a doorway, in the circles. The outer ring of stones will be broken, and there will be a stone path going up to the center of the wheel.

Likewise many medicine wheels have assorted other circles around the outside of the wheel, occasionally attached to spokes or the outer ring, and occasionally just seemingly floating free of the chief structure.

Chapter 10: Medicine Man

Synopsis

The primary function of these "medicine elders" (who are not constantly male) is to secure the help of the spirit world, including the Great Spirit, for the advantage of the total community.

The Healers

Occasionally the help sought-after might be for the sake of healing disease, healing the psyche, or the goal is to advance harmony between human groups or between humans & nature. So the term "medicine man/woman" isn't totally inappropriate, but it greatly oversimplifies and likewise skews the depiction of the individuals whose role in society complements that of the chief. These individuals are not the Native American equal of the Chinese "barefoot doctors", herbalists, nor of the emergency medical technicians who ride rescue vehicles.

To be acknowledged as the one who executes this function of bridging between the natural world and the spiritual world for the advantage of the community, that community must validate a person in his role. Medicine men and women learn through a medicine society or from one teacher.

The term "medicine people" is generally used in Native American communities, for instance, when Arwen Nuttall (Cherokee) of the National Museum of the American Indian publishes, "The knowledge owned by medicine people is privileged, and it frequently remains in particular families."

Native Americans tend to be rather reluctant to talk about issues about medicine or medicine people with non-Indians. In a few cultures, the individuals won't even discuss these issues with Indians from other tribes. In most tribes medicine elders are not expected to promote or introduce themselves per se. An inquiry to a Native individual about religious beliefs or ceremonies is frequently viewed with misgiving.

WRAPPING UP

Native-American medicine is classed as an indigenous healing tradition. As 80% of the World's population can't afford Western hi-tech medicine, indigenous customs collectively play a crucial global healthcare role - such so that the World Health Organization advocated that they be integrated into national healthcare policies and plans.

While Native-American healing reflects the diverseness of the many Native nations or tribes that have inhabited North America, basic themes exist not only between them but with a lot of the World's geographically diverse, ancient indigenous customs.

Printed in Great Britain
by Amazon